The Essential
Keto Diet For Women
Over 50

The Complete Guide To Ketogenic
Diet For People Over 50 With Some
Delicious Keto Friendly Recipes

Tiffany Johnson

TABLE OF CONTENTS

SNACKS RECIPES 57

VEGETABLES RECIPES 72

INTRODUCTION

Women looking for a quick and effective way to shed excess weight, get high blood sugar levels under control, reduce overall inflammation, and improve physical and mental energy will do their best by following a ketogenic diet plan. But there are special considerations women must take into account when they are beginning the keto diet.

A Ketogenic Diet is something that you should be starting with today for a better lifestyle if you are over 50. The ketogenic diet is more common in women than in men because of all the benefits it provides for dealing with the symptoms of menopause. Women who are experiencing menopause, or have already experienced it, have a clear idea of the troubles that come along with it. Menopause leads to fatigue, irritability and also increases weight. But the keto diet can help in controlling your body weight and also improve your physical well-being. Not sure from where or how to start with keto?

Being 50 years old or more is not bad. It is how we handle ourselves in this age that matters. Most of us would have just moved on and dealt with things as they would have arrived. That is no longer the case. It is quite literally survival of the fittest.

Do not try to work toward the lean body that many men sport. It is best for the overall function that women stay at twenty-two to twenty-six percent body fat. Our hormones will function best in this range, and we can't possibly work without our hormones. Like gymnasts and extreme athletes, very lean women will find their hormones no longer function or function at a less than optimal rate. And remember that the ideal weight may not be the right weight for you. Many women find that they perform their best when they are at their happy weight. If you find yourself fighting with yourself to lose the last few pounds you think you need to lose to have the perfect body, it may not be worth it. The struggle will affect your hormone function. Carefully observing the keto diet will allow your hormones to stabilize and regulate themselves back to their pre-obesity normal function.

As a woman, you know that sometimes your emotions get the better of you. It is true with your body, as you well know, and can be a major reason, women find it extremely difficult to lose weight the way they want to lose weight. We have been led to believe that not only can we do it all but that we must do it all. It gives many women extreme levels of pressure and can cause them to engage in emotional eating. Some women might have lowered self-worth feelings and may not feel they are entitled to the benefits of the keto diet, and turning to food relieves the feelings of inadequacy that we try to hide from the world.

The keto diet is naturally lower in calories if you follow the recommended levels of food intake. It is not necessary to try to restrict your intake of calories even further. All you need to do is only to eat until you are full and not one bite more. Besides losing weight, the keto diet aims to retrain your body on how to work properly. You will need to learn to trust your body and the signals it sends out to readjust to a proper way of eating.

Do not give up now as there will be quite a few days where you may think to yourself, "Why am I doing this?" and to answer that, focus on the goals you wish to achieve.

Whether you want to stay active, lose weight, look and feel better, or any of that, keto is your solution and a way of life that will ensure you get all you need.

BREAKFAST

1. Beef Taco Filling

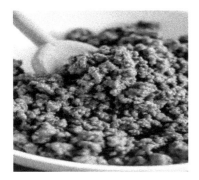

Preparation Time: 10 minutes

Cooking Time: 6 hours

Servings: 12

Ingredients:

- 1 lb. ground beef
- 10 oz... can tomato with green chilies
- 1 envelope taco seasoning

Directions:

1. Combine all ingredients and stir well.
2. Cover and cook on low.
3. Serve and enjoy.

Nutrition: Calories 75 Fat 2.4 g Carbs 0.9 g Sugar 0.6 g Protein 11.7 g Cholesterol 34 mg

2. Garlic Herb Pork

Preparation Time: 10 minutes

Cooking Time: 8 hours

Servings: 10

Ingredients:

- 3 lbs. pork shoulder roast, boneless and cut into 4 pieces
- 1/2 tbsp... cumin
- 1/2 tbsp... fresh oregano
- 2/3 cup grapefruit juice
- 6 garlic cloves
- Pepper and salt

Directions:

1. Add pork roast into the slow cooker. Season with pepper and salt.
2. Add garlic, cumin, oregano, and grapefruit juice into the blender and blend until smooth.
3. Pour blended mixture over pork and stir well.
4. Cover and cook on low.
5. Detach pork from slow cooker and shred
6. Take back shredded pork into the slow cooker and stir well.
7. Serve warm and enjoy.

Nutrition: Calories 359 Fat 27.8 g Carbs 2.1 g Sugar 1.1 g Protein 23.2 g

3. Garlic Thyme Lamb Chops

Preparation Time: 10 minutes

Cooking Time: 6 hours

Servings: 8

Ingredients:

- 8 lamb chops
- 1 tsp.... dried oregano
- 2 garlic cloves, minced
- 1/2 tsp.... dried thyme
- 1 medium onion, sliced
- Pepper and salt

Directions:

1. Add sliced onion into the slow cooker.
2. Combine together thyme, oregano, pepper, and salt. Rub over lamb chops.
3. Place lamb chops in slow cooker and top with garlic.
4. Pour 1/4 cup water around the lamb chops.
5. Cover and cook on low.
6. Serve and enjoy.

Nutrition: Calories 40 Fat 1.9 g Carbs 2.3 g Sugar 0.6 g Protein 3.4 g Cholesterol 0 mg

4. Pork Tenderloin

Preparation Time: 10 minutes

Cooking Time: 4 hours

Servings: 6

Ingredients:

- 1 1/2 lbs. pork tenderloin, trimmed and cut in half lengthwise
- 6 garlic cloves, chopped
- 1 oz... envelope dry onion soup mix
- 3/4 cup red wine
- 1 cup water
- Pepper and salt

Directions:

1. Place pork tenderloin into the slow cooker.
2. Pour red wine and water over pork.
3. Set dry onion soup mix on top of pork tenderloin.
4. Top with chopped garlic and season with pepper and salt.
5. Cover and cook on low.
6. Stir well and serve.

Nutrition: Calories 196 Fat 4 g Carbs 3.1 g Sugar 0.9 g Protein 29.9 g Cholesterol 83 mg

5. Tuna in Potatoes

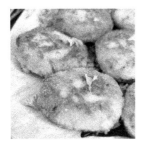

Preparation time: 16 minutes

Cooking time: 4 hours

Servings: 8

Ingredients:

- 4large potatoes
- 8oz. tuna, canned
- 1/2cup cream cheese
- 4oz. Cheddar cheese
- 1garlic clove
- 1teaspoon onion powder
- 1/2teaspoon salt
- 1teaspoon ground black pepper
- 1teaspoon dried dill

Directions:

1. Wash the potatoes carefully and cut them into the halves.

2. Wrap the potatoes in the foil and place in the slow cooker. Close the slow cooker lid and cook the potatoes on HIGH for 2 hours.

3. Meanwhile, peel the garlic clove and mince it. Combine the minced garlic clove with the cream cheese, tuna, salt, ground black pepper, onion powder, and dill.

4. Then shred Cheddar cheese and add it to the mixture.

5. Mix it carefully until homogenous.

6. When the time is over – remove the potatoes from the slow cooker and discard the foil only from the flat surface of the potatoes.

7. Then take the fork and mash the flesh of the potato halves gently. Add the tuna mixture in the potato halves and return them back in the slow cooker.

8. Cook the potatoes for 2 hours more on HIGH. Enjoy!

Nutrition: Calories 247, Fat 5.9, Fiber 4, Carbs 3.31, Protein 14

6. Banana Lunch Sandwiches

Preparation time: 15 minutes

Cooking time: 2 hours

Servings: 4

Ingredients:

- 2 bananas
- 8 oz. French toast slices, frozen
- 1tablespoon peanut butter
- 1/4teaspoon ground cinnamon
- 5oz. Cheddar cheese, sliced
- 1/4teaspoon turmeric

Directions:

1. Peel the bananas and slice them.
2. Spread the French toast slices with the peanut butter well. Combine the ground cinnamon with the turmeric and stir the mixture. Sprinkle the French toasts with the spice mixture.
3. Then make the layer of the sliced bananas on the toasts and add the sliced cheese.
4. Cover the toast with the second part of the toast to make the sandwich.
5. Place the banana sandwiches in the slow cooker and cook them on HIGH for 2 hours.
6. Serve the prepared banana sandwiches hot. Enjoy!

Nutrition: Calories 248, Fat 7.5, Fiber 2, Carbs 3.74 Protein 10

7. Parmesan Potato with Dill

Preparation time: 17 minutes

Cooking time: 4 hours

Servings: 5

Ingredients:

- 1-pound small potato
- 1/2 cup fresh dill
- 7 oz. Parmesan
- 1teaspoon rosemary
- 1teaspoon thyme
- 1cup water
- 1/4 teaspoon chili flakes
- 3tablespoon cream
- 1teaspoon salt

Directions:

1. Peel the potatoes and put them in the slow cooker.
2. Add water, salt, thyme, rosemary, and chili flakes.
3. Close the slow cooker lid and cook the potato for 2 hours on HIGH.
4. Meanwhile, shred Parmesan cheese and chop the fresh dill. When the time is done, sprinkle the potato with the cream and fresh dill. Stir it carefully.

5. Add shredded Parmesan cheese and close the slow cooker lid. Cook the potato on HIGH for 2 hours more.

6. Then open the slow cooker lid and do not stir the potato anymore. Gently transfer the dish to the serving plates. Enjoy!

Nutrition: Calories 235, Fat 3.9, Fiber 2, Carbs 2.26, Protein 1

8. Light Taco Soup

Preparation time: 24 minutes

Cooking time: 7 hours

Servings: 5

Ingredients:

- 7oz. ground chicken
- 1/2teaspoon sesame oil
- 3cup vegetable stock
- 3oz. yellow onion
- 1cup tomato, canned
- 3tomatoes
- 5 oz. corn kernels
- 1jalapeno pepper, sliced
- 1/2cup white beans, drained
- 3tablespoon taco seasoning
- 1/4teaspoon salt
- 3 oz. black olives, sliced
- 5 corn tortillas, for serving

Directions:

1. Peel the onion and dice it. Chop the fresh and canned tomatoes.

2. Place the ground chicken, sesame oil, vegetable stock, diced onion, chopped tomatoes, sliced black olives, sliced jalapeno pepper, and corn in the slow cooker.

3. Add the white beans, taco seasoning, and salt.

4. Stir the soup mixture gently and close the slow cooker lid.

5. Cook the soup for 7 hours on LOW. Meanwhile, cut the corn tortillas into the strips and bake them in the preheated to 365 F oven for 10 minutes.

6. When the soup is cooked, ladle it into the serving bowls and sprinkle with the baked corn tortilla strips. Enjoy!

Nutrition: Calories 328, Fat 9.6, Fiber 10, Carbs 4.19, Protein 18

9. Slow Cooker Risotto

Preparation time: 20 minutes

Cooking time: 3 hours 30 minutes

Servings: 6

Ingredients:

- 7 oz. Parmigiano-Reggiano
- 2cup chicken broth
- 1teaspoon olive oil
- 1onion, chopped
- 1/2cup green peas
- 1garlic clove, peeled and sliced
- 2cups long grain rice
- 1/4cup dry wine
- 1teaspoon salt
- 1teaspoon ground black pepper
- 1carrot, chopped
- 1cup beef broth

Directions:

1. Spray a skillet with olive oil.
2. Add the chopped onion and carrot and roast the vegetables for 3 minutes on the medium heat. Then put the seared vegetables in the slow cooker. Toss the long

grain rice in the remaining oil and sauté for 1 minute on the high heat.

3. Add the roasted long grain rice and sliced garlic in the slow cooker.

4. Add green peas, dry wine, salt, ground black pepper, and beef broth. After this, add the chicken broth and stir the mixture gently. Close the slow cooker lid and cook the risotto for 3 hours.

5. Then stir the risotto gently.

6. Shred Parmigiano-Reggiano and sprinkle over the risotto. Close the slow cooker lid and cook the dish for 30 minutes more. Enjoy the prepared risotto immediately!

Nutrition: Calories 268, Fat 3, Fiber 4, Carbs 3.34, Protein 7

10. <u>Lemon Orzo</u>

Preparation time: 20 minutes

Cooking time: 2 hours 30 minutes

Servings: 5

Ingredients:

- 4oz. shallot
- 7oz. orzo
- 2cup chicken stock
- 1teaspoon paprika
- 1teaspoon ground black pepper
- 1teaspoon salt
- 1lemon
- 1/4cup cream
- 2yellow sweet pepper
- 1cup baby spinach

Directions:

1. Chop the shallot and place it in the slow cooker.
2. Add the chicken stock and paprika. Sprinkle the mixture with the ground black pepper and salt. Stir it gently and cook on HIGH for 30 minutes.
3. Meanwhile, grate the zest from the lemon and squeeze the juice. Add the lemon zest and juice in the slow cooker and stir it. After this, chop the baby spinach.

4. Add it into the slow cooker. Remove the seeds from the yellow sweet peppers and chop into tiny pieces. Add the chopped peppers to the slow cooker.

5. Add orzo and heavy cream. Stir the mass carefully and close the slow cooker lid. Cook the dish for 2 hours on LOW. Mix the dish gently. Enjoy!

Nutrition: Calories 152, Fat 4, Fiber 3, Carbs 2.79, Protein 7

11. <u>Veggie Bean Stew</u>

Preparation time: 20 minutes

Cooking time: 7 hours

Servings: 8

Ingredients:

- 1/2cup barley
- 1cup black beans
- 1/4cup red beans
- 2carrots
- 1cup onion, chopped
- 1cup tomato juice
- 2potatoes
- 1teaspoon salt
- 1teaspoon ground black pepper
- 4cups water
- 4oz. tofu
- 1teaspoon garlic powder
- 1cup fresh cilantro

Directions:

1. Place barley, black beans, and red beans in the slow cooker vessel.

2. Add chopped onion, tomato juice, salt, ground black pepper, and garlic powder. After this, add water and close the slow cooker lid.

3. Cook the dish for 4 hours on HIGH.

4. Meanwhile, peel the carrots and cut them into the strips. Peel the potatoes and chop.

5. Add the carrot strips and chopped potatoes in the slow cooker after 4 hours of cooking.

6. Chop the fresh cilantro and add it in the slow cooker too.

7. Stir the mix and close the slow cooker lid. Cook the stew for 3 hours more on LOW.

8. Serve the prepared dish immediately or keep it in the fridge, not more than 3 days. Enjoy!

Nutrition: Calories 207, Fat 3.5, Fiber 8, Carbs 3.67, Protein 8

12. Carrot Soup with Cardamom

Preparation time: 18 minutes

Cooking time: 12 hours

Servings: 9

Ingredients:

- 1pound carrot
- 1teaspoon ground cardamom
- 1/4teaspoon nutmeg
- 1teaspoon salt
- 3tablespoons fresh parsley
- 1teaspoon honey
- 1teaspoon marjoram
- 5cups chicken stock
- 1/2cup yellow onion, chopped
- 1teaspoon butter

Directions:

1. Toss the butter in a pan and add chopped onion.
2. Chop the carrot and add it to the pan too.
3. Roast the vegetables for 5 minutes on the low heat. After this, place the roasted vegetables in the slow cooker. Add ground cardamom, nutmeg, salt, marjoram, and chicken stock.

4. Close the slow cooker lid and cook the soup for 12 hours on LOW.

5. Chop the fresh parsley.

6. When the time is over, blend the soup with a hand blender until you get a smooth texture. Then ladle the soup into the serving bowls.

7. Sprinkle the prepared soup with the chopped fresh parsley and honey. Enjoy the soup immediately!

Nutrition: Calories 80 Fat 2.7 Fiber 2, Carbs 1.19 Protein 4

13. Cod Chowder

Preparation time: 20 minutes

Cooking time: 3 hours

Servings: 6

Ingredients:

- yellow onion
- 10oz. cod
- 3oz. bacon, sliced
- 1teaspoon sage
- 5oz. potatoes
- 1carrot, grated
- 5cups water
- 1tablespoon almond milk
- 1teaspoon ground coriander
- 1teaspoon salt

Directions:

1. Peel the onion and chop it.

2. Put the chopped onion and grated carrot in the slow cooker bowl. Add the sage, almond milk, ground coriander, and water. After this, chop the cod into the 6 pieces.

3. Add the fish in the slow cooker bowl too. Then chop the sliced bacon and peel the potatoes.

4. Cut the potatoes into the cubes.

5. Add the Ingredients: in the slow cooker bowl and close the slow cooker lid.

6. Cook the chowder for 3 hours on HIGH. Ladle the prepared cod chowder in the serving bowls.

7. Sprinkle the dish with the chopped parsley if desired. Enjoy!

Nutrition: Calories 108 Fat 4.5 Fiber 2, Carbs 3.02 Protein 10

14. Sweet Corn Pilaf

Preparation time: 21 minutes

Cooking time: 8 hours

Servings: 5

Ingredients:

- 2cups rice
- 1cup sweet corn, frozen
- 6oz. chicken fillet
- 1sweet red pepper
- 1yellow sweet pepper
- 1/2cup green peas, frozen
- 1carrot
- 4cups chicken stock
- 2tablespoon chopped almonds
- 1teaspoon olive oil
- 1teaspoon salt
- 1teaspoon ground white pepper

Directions:

1. Peel the carrot and cut into the small cubes.
2. Combine the carrot cubes with the frozen sweet corn and green peas.
3. After this, place the vegetable mixture in the slow cooker vessel.

4. Add the rice, chicken stock, olive oil, salt, and ground white pepper.

5. After this, cut the chicken fillet into the strips and add the meat to the rice mixture.

6. Chop all the sweet peppers and add them in the slow cooker too.

7. Close the slow cooker lid and cook the pilaf for 8 hours on LOW.

8. When the pilaf is cooked, stir it gently and sprinkle with the almonds. Mix the dish carefully again. Serve it immediately. Enjoy!

Nutrition: Calories 390, Fat 18.6, Fiber 13, Carbs 4.7, Protein 18

DINNER

15. Pepper Jalapeno Low Carb Soup

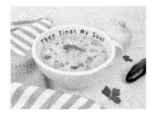

Preparation Time: 10 minutes

Cooking Time: 7 hours

Servings: 8

Ingredients:

- 1/4 teaspoon Paprika
- 1/2 teaspoon Pepper
- 1/2 chopped onion
- 1/2 teaspoon Xanthan gum
- 1/2 chopped green pepper
- 1/2 cup heavy whipping cream
- 1/2 lb. Cooked & crumbled bacon
- 3/4 cup cheddar cheese
- 3/4 cup Monterrey jack cheese
- teaspoon Salt
- 1 teaspoon Cumin
- 1 & 1/2-pounds chicken breasts, boneless
- Minced garlic cloves
- Seeded & chopped jalapenos
- 1tbsp. Butter

- 3 cups chicken broth
- Oz. Cream cheese

Directions:

1. Dissolve the butter, then cook the green peppers, seasoning, jalapenos, and onions until translucent in a medium-sized pan.

2. Scoop the mixture into the crockpot, then add in the chicken broth and breast.

3. Cover the crockpot, then cook for 3-4 hours on high or 6-7 hours on a low setting.

4. Separate the chicken, and shred it, then return it into the crockpot.

5. Put in the heavy whipping cream, cream cheese, remaining cheeses, bacon, then stir until the cheese melts.

6. Sprinkle the soup with xanthan gum to thicken, then allow it to simmer uncovered on low for 10 minutes.

7. Serve, then top with cheddar cheese, bacon, or jalapenos and enjoy.

Nutrition: Calories: 240 Carbs: 1g Fat: 20g Protein: 11g

16. Lean Beef & Mixed Veggies Soup

Preparation Time: 8 minutes

Cooking Time: 6 hours

Servings: 6

Ingredients:

- 1/2 teaspoon Garlic salt, if desired
- Peeled small onion
- 1 diced small green pepper
- 1 teaspoon Garlic & herb seasoning
- 1 small zucchini, sliced into rounds
- 1 can of rinsed & drained cannellini beans
- 1 small yellow squash, sliced into rounds
- 1 (14 1/2 ounces) can diced roasted tomatoes
- 1 & 1/2-pounds beef stew meat
- 1-2 teaspoon Ground pepper
- 1-3 bay leaves
- Cups of frozen mixed vegetables
- Cups low salt beef broth
- Peeled & chopped garlic cloves

Directions:

1. Add all the ingredients except the zucchini cannellini beans, mixed vegetables, and yellow squash into the crockpot.

2. Cover the pot, then cook on high for 4 hours.

3. After 4 hours, add in the zucchini, cannellini beans, yellow squash, and mixed vegetables.

4. Season to taste, and cook for an extra 2 hours on high.

5. Once done, stir, then serve and enjoy.

Nutrition: Calories: 50 Carbs: 1g Fat: 0g Protein: 2g

17. Sumptuous Ham and Lentil Consommé

Preparation Time: 15 minutes

Cooking Time: 11 hours

Servings: 6

Ingredients:

- 8 teaspoons tomato sauce
- Cup onion, diced
- 1 cup dried lentils
- 1 cup of water
- 1 cup celery, chopped
- 1/2 teaspoon dried basil
- 32 ounces' chicken broth
- 1 cup carrots, diced
- 1/4 teaspoon dried thyme
- 1/4 teaspoon black pepper
- Cloves garlic, minced
- 1/2 teaspoon dried oregano
- 1 1/2 cups diced cooked ham
- 1 bay leaf

Directions:

1. Put all your fixing into your slow cooker and mix very well to blend well.

2. Cook within 11 hours, low heat settings. Remove your bay leaf before serving it.

Nutrition: Calories: 194 Carbs: 2.1g Fat: 4g Protein: 20g

18. Crock Pot Pork Stew with Tapioca

Preparation Time: 15 minutes

Cooking Time: 10 hours

Servings: 6

Ingredients:

- 3 tablespoons quick-cooking tapioca
- Tablespoon vegetable oil
- 1/4 teaspoon pepper
- 1 large onion, chopped
- 1 1/2 lb. Pork stew meat, cut into bite-size pieces
- Teaspoons Worcestershire sauce
- 1 stalk celery, chopped
- Carrots, sliced
- 1 tablespoon beef bouillon granules
- Red potatoes, cubes
- 3 cups vegetable juice

Directions:

1. Heat your oil over medium-high heat using a Dutch oven; brown your beef on all sides.

2. Mix your browned beef with all other ingredients in the crockpot.

3. Cover and cook on low heat settings for 9-10 hours.

Nutrition: Calories: 190 Carbs: 0g Fat: 10g Protein: 23g

19. Beef Barley Vegetable Soup

Preparation Time: 15 minutes

Cooking Time: 8 hours

Servings: 10

Ingredients:

- Package frozen mixed vegetables
- Ground black pepper to taste
- 1 beef chuck roast
- 1 onion, chopped
- Salt to taste
- 1/2 cup barley
- 4 cups of water
- 1 can chop stewed tomatoes
- 1 bay leaf
- Stalks celery, chopped
- 1/4 teaspoon ground black pepper
- Carrots, chopped
- 4 cubes beef bouillon cube
- 2 tablespoons oil
- 1 tablespoon white sugar

Directions:

1. Season your beef with salt, adding bay leaf and barley in the last hour; cook your beef in your slow cooker for 8 hours or until tender.
2. Set your beef aside; keep your broth also aside.
3. Stir fry your onion, celery, carrots, and frozen vegetable mix until soft.

4. Add your bouillon cubes, pepper, water, salt, beef mixture, barley mixture, chopped stewed tomatoes, and broth.
5. Bring to boiling point and simmer at lowered heat for 20 minutes.

Nutrition: Calories: 69 Carbs: 1g Fat: 2g Protein: 5g

20. Delicious Chicken Soup with Lemongrass

Preparation Time: 5 minutes

Cooking Time: 8 hours

Servings: 10

Ingredients:

- 1 stalk of lemongrass, cut into big chunks
- 1 whole chicken
- 1 Tablespoon of salt
- 5 thick slices of fresh ginger
- 20 fresh basil leaves (10 -slow cooker; 10 -spices)
- 1 lime

Directions:

1. Put your lemongrass, ginger, 10 basil leaves, salt, and chicken into the slow cooker.
2. Fill the slow cooker up with water. Boil the chicken mixture for 480 - 600 minutes.
3. Scoop the soup into a bowl and adjust your salt to taste. Juice in the lime to taste and spice up with the chopped basil leaves.

Nutrition: Calories: 105 Carbs: 1g Fat: 2g Protein: 15g

21. Delicious Bacon Cheese Potato Soup

Preparation Time: 15 minutes

Cooking Time: 10 hours

Servings: 8

Ingredients:

- 3 lb. large baking potatoes, peeled, cut into 1/2-inch cubes
- 1/4 cup chopped fresh chives
- 8 slices bacon, diced
- carton fat-free reduced-sodium chicken broth, divided
- 1/2 cup milk
- 1 onion, finely chopped
- 1 pkg. Shredded Triple Cheddar Cheese, divided
- 1/2 cup Sour Cream
- 2 tablespoons flour

Directions:

1. Stir fry bacon over medium heat in a large skillet. Remove bacon with your slotted spoon and leave the drippings in the skillet.
2. Stir fry your onions in the skillet for few minutes until it is soft and crisp. Add in your flour and cook for 1 minute, stirring it frequently.
3. Add 1 cup of your chicken broth and cook for 2-3 minutes or until sauce is thick and simmers. Pour the sauce into your slow cooker.

4. Add your remaining chicken broth and potatoes and cook with a slow cooker cover for 8-10 hours on low heat settings.
5. Transfer 4 cups of your potatoes in a bowl and mash it until smooth, adding 1.5 cups of cheese to the remaining mixture in the slow cooker; stir until melted.
6. Stir your mashed potatoes into the slow cooker with milk added and cook again within 5 minutes with the lid.
7. Microwave your bacon in a microwavable plate within 30 seconds or until heated.
8. Serve your soup with bacon, using sour cream, chives, and remaining cheese as toppings.

Nutrition: Calories: 100 Carbs: 1.8g Fat: 0g Protein: 2g

22. Tasty Tomato Soup with Parmesan and Basil

Preparation Time: 15 minutes

Cooking Time: 3 hours

Servings: 6

Ingredients:

- 28 oz. of tomatoes, chopped
- 1/2 cup heavy cream
- 1/2 cup grated parmesan cheese
- 10-12 large basil leaves
- 3 tablespoons chopped garlic
- 2-3 Servings: of Erythritol
- 1/2 tablespoon dried thyme
- 1/4 teaspoon of red pepper flakes
- Tablespoon onion powder

Directions:

1. Add all ingredients except your parmesan and heavy cream to your crockpot and cook on high heat for 3 hours.
2. Add your cheese and cream and stir. Adjust seasoning to taste. Enjoy.

Nutrition: Calories: 110 Carbs: 1.6g Fat: 3g Protein: 5g

23. Chicken & Tortilla Soup

Preparation Time: 7 minutes

Cooking Time: 2 hours & 10 minutes

Servings: 6

Ingredients:

- 1 diced sweet onion
- 1 teaspoon cumin
- 1teaspoon chili powder
- 1 neatly chopped cilantro bunch
- 1 (28 ounces) can diced tomatoes
- 1-2 cups water
- 2 cups celery, chopped
- 2 cups carrots, shredded
- 2 tablespoons tomato paste
- 2 diced & de-seeded jalapenos
- 2 big skinned chicken breasts, sliced into 1/2" strips
- 4 minced garlic cloves
- 32 ounces' organic chicken broth
- Olive oil
- Sea salt & fresh cracked pepper, as desired

Directions:

1. Pour a dash of olive oil, 1/4 cup of chicken broth, the garlic, onions, pepper, jalapeno, and sea salt into a Dutch oven and cook over medium-high heat until soft.
2. Transfer the mixture into the crockpot and ass in the remaining ingredients and cook for 2 hours on low settings.

3. Shred the chicken, then top with the cilantro, avocado slices and enjoy.

Nutrition: Calories: 130 Carbs: 1.6g Fat: 5g Protein: 8g

24. Chicken Chile Verde

Preparation Time: 12 minutes

Cooking Time: 6 hours

Servings: 9

Ingredients:

- 1/4 teaspoon sea salt
- 2 pounds chopped boneless chicken.
- 3 tablespoons divided butter
- 3 tablespoons neatly chopped & divided cilantro
- 5 minced & divided garlic cloves
- 1 extra tablespoon cilantro, to garnish
- 1 1/2 cups salsa Verde

Directions:

1. Dissolve 2 tablespoons of butter in the slow cooker on high.
2. Add in 4 of the garlic along with 2 tablespoons cilantro, then stir.
3. Use a stovetop, melt 1 tablespoon butter in a big fry pan over medium-high heat, and add 1 tablespoon minced garlic and cilantro.
4. Put in the chopped chicken, then sear until all the sides are browned but not cooked through.
5. Add the cilantro, garlic, and butter mixture with browned chicken into the crockpot.
6. Pour in the salsa Verde and stir together.
7. Cover the crockpot and cook on high settings for 2 hours, then reduce to a low setting for 3-4 extra hours.

8. Serve the chicken Verde in a lettuce cup or over cauliflower rice.

Nutrition: Calories: 140 Carbs: 5 g Fat: 4g Protein: 18g

25. Cauliflower & Ham Potato Stew

Preparation Time: 5 minutes

Cooking Time: 4 hours

Servings: 6

Ingredients:

- 1/4 teaspoon salt
- 1/4 cup heavy cream
- 1/2 teaspoon onion powder
- 1/2 teaspoon garlic powder
- 3 cups diced ham
- 4 garlic cloves
- 8 oz. grated cheddar cheese
- 14 1/2 oz. chicken broth
- 16 oz. bag frozen cauliflower florets
- A dash of pepper

Directions:

1. Put all the items except the cauliflower inside the crockpot and mix.
2. Cover the crockpot, then cook for 4 hours on a high setting.
3. Once done, add in the cauliflower and cook for an extra 30 minutes on high. Serve and enjoy.

Nutrition: Calories: 71 Carbs: 2g Fat: 4g Protein: 6g

26. Beef Dijon

Preparation Time: 15 minutes

Cooking Time: 5 hours

Servings: 4

Ingredients:

- 6 oz. Small round steaks
- 2 tbsp. of each:
- Steak seasoning - to taste
- Avocado oil
- Peanut oil
- Balsamic vinegar/dry sherry
- Large chopped green onions/small chopped onions for the garnish - extra
- 1/4 c. whipping cream
- 1cup. fresh cremini mushrooms - sliced
- 1tbsp. Dijon mustard

Directions:

1. Warm up the oils using the high heat setting on the stove top. Flavor each of the steaks with pepper and arrange to a skillet.
2. Cook two to three minutes per side until done.
3. Place into the slow cooker. Pour in the skillet drippings, half of the mushrooms, and the onions.
4. Cook on the low setting for four hours.

5. When the cooking time is done, scoop out the onions, mushrooms, and steaks to a serving platter.
6. In a separate dish - whisk together the mustard, balsamic vinegar, whipping cream, and the steak drippings from the slow cooker.
7. Empty the gravy into a gravy server and pour over the steaks.
8. Enjoy with some brown rice, riced cauliflower, or potatoes.

Nutrition: Calories: 535 Carbs: 5.0 g Fat: 40 g Protein: 39 g

27. Chipotle Baracoa

Preparation Time: 20 minutes

Cooking Time: 4 hours

Servings: 9

Ingredients:

- 1/2 cup beef/chicken broth
- 4tsp chilies
- 1lb. chuck roast/beef brisket
- Minced garlic cloves
- 2tbsp.Lime juice
- 2tbsp.Apple cider vinegar
- 1tsps. of each:
- 1tsps. Sea salt
- 2 tsps. Cumin
- 1 tbsp. dried oregano
- 1 tsp. black pepper
- whole bay leaves
- Optional: 1/2 t. ground cloves

Directions:

1. Mix the chilies in the sauce, and add the broth, garlic, ground cloves, pepper, cumin, salt, vinegar, and lime juice in a blender, mixing until smooth.

2. Chop the beef into two-inch chunks and toss it in the slow cooker. Empty the puree on top. Toss in the two bay leaves.

3. Cook four to six hrs. On the high setting or eight to ten using the low setting.

4. Dispose of the bay leaves when the meat is done.

5. Shred and stir into the juices to simmer for five to ten minutes.

Nutrition: Calories: 242 Net Carbs: 2 g Fat: 11 g Protein: 32 g

28. Cube Steak

Preparation Time: 15 minutes

Cooking Time: 8 hours

Servings: 8

Ingredients:

- 28 oz. Cubed steaks
- 1 3/4 t. adobo seasoning/garlic salt
- 1 can (8 oz.) tomato sauce
- 1 c. water
- Black pepper to taste
- 1/2 med. onion
- 1 small red pepper
- 1/3 c. green pitted olives
- 2 tbsp. brine

Directions:

1. Slice the peppers and onions into 1/4-inch strips.
2. Sprinkle the steaks with the pepper and garlic salt as needed and place them in the cooker.
3. Fold in the peppers and onion along with the water, sauce, and olives (with the liquid/brine from the jar).
4. Close the lid. Prepare using the low-temperature setting for eight hours.

Nutrition: Calories: 154 Carbs: 4 g Protein: 23.5 g Fat: 5.5 g

SNACKS RECIPES

29. Chicken Spinach Meatballs

Preparation Time: 5 minutes

Cooking Time: 15 minutes

Servings: 15

Ingredients:

- 1-pound ground chicken
- 1/2 cup frozen spinach
- 1 egg
- 1/2 cup shredded pepper jack cheese
- 1-ounce cream cheese
- 1 teaspoon salt
- 1/4 teaspoon pepper
- 1/4 teaspoon garlic powder
- 1/4 teaspoon dried parsley
- 1 cup water
- 2 tablespoons coconut oil

Directions:

1. Mix all ingredients except water and coconut oil in large mixing bowl. Roll into 12 balls. Pour water into Instant Pot and place steamer rack in bottom. Place

meatballs on rack. (You may have to cook in two batches.) Click lid closed.

2. Press the Manual button and adjust time for 10 minutes. When timer beeps, allow a 5-minute natural release. Quick-release the remaining pressure. Remove rack with meatballs and set aside. Pour out water and replace inner pot.

3. Press the Sauté button and add coconut oil to Instant Pot®. Once oil is heated, add meatballs until browned and crispy.

Nutrition: Calories: 216 Protein: 17.3 g Fiber: 0.4 g Fat: 14.9 g Sodium: 528 mg Carbohydrates: 1.2 g Sugar: 0.3 g

30. Easy Tomato Sauce

Preparation Time: 5 minutes

Cooking Time: 30 minutes

Servings: 21

Ingredients:

- 3 tablespoons butter
- 1/2 medium onion, finely diced
- 1 clove garlic, finely minced
- 2 (6-ounce) cans tomato paste
- 2 cups Chicken Broth (see recipe in Chapter 3)
- 1 teaspoon fresh parsley
- 1/2 teaspoon oregano
- 1/2 teaspoon basil

Directions:

1. Press the Sauté button. Sauté onion until translucent. Add garlic and sauté for 30 seconds. Press the Cancel button.

2. Add remaining ingredients to Instant Pot and stir. Click lid closed. Press the Manual button and adjust time for 30 minutes. When timer beeps, quick-release the pressure.

Nutrition: Calories: 65 Protein: 1.9 g Fiber: 1.5 g Fat: 3.6 g Sodium: 270 mg Carbohydrates: 2.7 g Sugar: 4.4 g

31. Bacon Broccoli Salad

Preparation Time: 10 minutes

Cooking Time: 10 minutes

Servings: 4

Ingredients:

- 6 slices bacon
- 4 cups fresh broccoli, chopped
- 1/4 cup mayo
- 3 tablespoons Thai chili sauce
- 2 tablespoons pepitas

Directions:

1. Press the Sauté button and add bacon to Instant Pot. Cook bacon until crisp.

2. When bacon is cooked, remove and place on paper towel until cool. Add broccoli into bacon grease and stir-fry for 3 minutes until just beginning to soften. Press the Cancel button.

3. Remove broccoli and place in large bowl to set aside. In small bowl, mix mayo and chili sauce. Add sauce mixture to large bowl. Crumble bacon over bowl and toss. Sprinkle pepitas on top to serve. Serve warm or cold.

Nutrition: Calories: 319 Protein: 7.9 g Fiber: 0.4 g Fat: 26.2 g Sodium: 463 mg Carbohydrates: 3.7 g Sugar: 5.0 g

32. Classic Deviled Eggs

This classic party dish is a perfect keto snack. It's loaded with fats and protein to keep you going. Feel free to customize it with your favorite flavors such as bacon, or simply enjoy it as is.

Preparation Time: 15 minutes

Cooking Time: 8 minutes

Servings: 6

Ingredients:

- 6 eggs
- 1 cup water
- 1/4 cup mayo
- 1/2 teaspoon salt
- 1/8 teaspoon pepper
- 1/2 teaspoon yellow mustard
- 1/4 teaspoon paprika

Directions:

1. Place eggs on steamer basket and add to Instant Pot. Pour water into pot and click lid closed. Press the Egg button and adjust time for 8 minutes.

2. When timer beeps, quick-release the pressure and remove steamer basket. Place eggs in cold water and peel when cooled. Slice eggs in half lengthwise.

3. Remove yolks and set egg whites aside. Place yolks, mayo, salt, pepper, and mustard in food processor and blend until smooth. (Alternatively, press with fork until all ingredients are smooth.) Place filling into egg whites. Sprinkle with paprika and refrigerate at least 30 minutes or until chilled.

Nutrition: Calories: 268 Protein: 12.8 g Fiber: 0.1 g Fat: 22.1 g Sodium: 650 mg Carbohydrates: 1.0 g Sugar: 0.5 g

33. Blackened Chicken Bites and Ranch

Preparation Time: 5 minutes

Cooking Time: 15 minutes

Servings: 1

Ingredients:

- 2 ounces boneless, skinless chicken breast, cubed
- 1/4 teaspoon dried thyme
- 1/4 teaspoon paprika
- 1/4 teaspoon pepper
- 1/4 teaspoon garlic powder
- 3 tablespoons coconut oil
- 1/2 cup ranch dressing
- 2 tablespoons hot sauce

Directions:

1. Toss chicken pieces in seasonings. Press the Sauté button and add coconut oil to Instant Pot. Sear chicken until dark golden brown and thoroughly cooked.

2. To make sauce, remove chicken from Instant Pot and press the Cancel button. Pour ranch and hot sauce into Instant Pot. Use wooden spoon to scrape any seasoning from bottom of pot. Heat on Keep Warm for 5 minutes. Pour into small bowl for serving. Serve chicken bites warm with dipping sauce.

Nutrition: Calories: 228 Protein: 6.8 g Fiber: 0.3 g Fat: 21.4 g Sodium: 135 mg Carbohydrates: 1.0 g Sugar: 0.2 g

34. Savory Snack Mix

Preparation Time: 5 minutes

Cooking Time: 2 hours

Servings: 6

Ingredients:

- 2 cups whole almonds
- 2 cups pork rinds
- 1/2 cup pecans
- 4 tablespoons butter
- 1 teaspoon chili powder
- 1/2 teaspoon garlic powder
- 1/8 teaspoon cayenne

Nutrition: Calories: 321 Protein: 10.4 g Fiber: 5.2 g Fat: 27.8 g Sodium: 75 mg Carbohydrates: 1.4 g Sugar: 1.8 grams

35. **Pickled Jalapeño and Bacon Dip**

Preparation Time: 3 minutes

Cooking Time: 3 minutes

Servings: 6

Ingredients:

- 1/2 cup pickled jalapeños
- 1/2 cup mayo
- 1 clove garlic, finely minced
- 8 ounces' cream cheese
- 1/2 cup cooked crumbled bacon
- 1/2 cup Chicken Broth (see recipe in Chapter 3)

Directions:

1. Add all ingredients to Instant Pot. Click lid closed. Adjust time for 3 minutes. Quick-release the pressure when timer beeps.

Nutrition: Calories: 354 Protein: 8.2 g Fiber: 0.6 g Fat: 29.9 g Sodium: 614 mg Carbohydrates: 1.8 g Sugar: 6.7 g

36. <u>Sweet Snack Mix</u>

Preparation Time: 5 minutes

Cooking Time: 2 hours

Servings: 6

Ingredients:

- 2 cups pork rinds
- 1 cup pecans
- 1/2 cup almonds
- 1/2 cup flaked unsweetened coconut
- 4 tablespoons butter
- 1/2 cup powdered Erythritol
- 2 egg whites
- 1/2 teaspoon cinnamon
- 2 teaspoons vanilla extract
- 1/4 cup low-carb chocolate chips

Directions:

2. Break pork rinds into bite-sized pieces and place into Instant Pot. Press the Sauté button and add pecans, almonds, coconut flakes, and butter. Cook 2–4 minutes until butter is completely melted. Press the Cancel button.

3. In medium bowl, whip Erythritol, egg whites, cinnamon, and vanilla until soft peaks form. Slowly add to Instant Pot. Gently fold mixture into ingredients

already in pot. Place slow cooker lid on pot and press the Slow Cook button. Adjust time for 2 hours. Stir every 20–30 minutes.

4. When mixture is dry and crunchy, place on parchment-lined baking sheet to cool. Once cooled fully, sprinkle with chocolate chips and store in sealed container.

Nutrition: Calories: 274 Protein: 6.4 g Fiber: 3.4 g Sugar Alcohols: 12.5 g Fat: 23.9 g Sodium: 80 mg Carbohydrates: 5 g Sugar: 1.3 g

37. Cheesy Zucchini Triangles with Garlic Mayo Dip

Preparation Time: 20 minutes

Cooking Time: 30 minutes

Servings: 4

Ingredients:

- Garlic Mayo Dip:
- cup crème Fraiche
- 1/3 cup mayonnaise
- 1/4 tsp. sugar-free maple syrup
- 1 garlic clove, pressed
- 1/2 tsp. vinegar
- Salt and black pepper to taste
- Cheesy Zucchini Triangles:
- 2 large zucchinis, grated
- 1egg
- 1/4 cup almond flour
- 1/4 tsp. paprika powder
- 3/4 tsp. dried mixed herbs
- 1/4 tsp. swerve sugar
- 1/2 cup grated mozzarella cheese

Directions:

1. Start by making the dip; in a medium bowl, mix the crème Fraiche, mayonnaise, maple syrup, garlic, vinegar, salt, and black pepper.

2. Cover the bowl with a plastic wrap and refrigerate while you make the zucchinis.

3. Let the oven preheat at 400F. And line a baking tray with greaseproof paper. Set aside.

4. Put the zucchinis in a cheesecloth and press out as much liquid as possible.

5. Pour the zucchinis in a bowl.

6. Add the egg, almond flour, paprika, dried mixed herbs, and swerve sugar.

7. Mix well and spread the mixture on the baking tray into a round pizza-like piece with 1-inch thickness.

8. Let it bake for 25 minutes.

9. Reduce the oven's heat to 350°F/175°C, take out the tray, and sprinkle the zucchini with the mozzarella cheese.

10. Let it melt in the oven.

11. Remove afterward, set aside to cool for 5 minutes, and then slice the snacks into triangles.

12. Serve immediately with the garlic mayo dip.

Nutrition: Calories: 286 Fat: 11.4g Fiber: 8.4g Carbohydrates: 4.3 g Protein: 10.1g

VEGETABLES RECIPES

38. Mexican Casserole with Black Beans

Preparation Time: 20 minutes

Cooking Time: 20 minutes

Servings: 6

Ingredients:

- 2 cups of minced garlic cloves
- 2 cups of Monterey Jack and cheddar
- 3/4 cup of salsa
- 2 1/2 cups chopped red pepper
- 2 teaspoons ground cumin
- 2 cans black beans
- 12 corn tortillas
- 2chopped tomatoes
- 1/2 cup of sliced black olives
- 2 cups of chopped onion

Directions:

1. Let the oven heat to 350F.
2. Place a large pot over medium heat.
3. Pour the onion, garlic, pepper, cumin, salsa, and black beans in the pot — Cook the ingredients for 3 minutes, stirring frequently.

4. Arrange the tortillas in the baking dish.

5. Ensure they are well spaced and even overlapping the dish if necessary.

6. Spread half of the bean's mixture on the tortillas. Sprinkle with the cheddar.

7. Repeat the process across the tortillas until everything is well stuffed.

8. Cover the baking dish with foil paper and place in the oven.

9. Bake it for 15 minutes. Remove from the oven to cool down a bit.

10. Garnish the casserole with olives and tomatoes

Nutrition: Calories: 325 Fat: 9.4g Fiber: 11.2g Carbohydrates: 3.1 g Protein: 12.6g

39. Baked Zucchini Gratin

Preparation Time: 25 minutes

Cooking Time: 30 minutes

Servings: 2

Ingredients:

- 1large zucchini, cut into 1/4-inch-thick slices
- Pink Himalayan salt
- 1-ounce Brie cheese, rind trimmed off
- 1 tablespoon butter
- Freshly ground black pepper
- 1/3 cup shredded Gruyere cheese
- 1/4 cup crushed pork rinds

Directions:

1. Preheat the oven to 400°F.

2. When the zucchini has been "weeping" for about 30 minutes, in a small saucepan over medium-low heat, heat the Brie and butter, occasionally stirring, until the cheese has melted.

3. The mixture is thoroughly combined for about 2 minutes.

4. Arrange the zucchini in an 8-inch baking dish, so the zucchini slices are overlapping a bit.

5. Season with pepper.

6. Pour the Brie mixture over the zucchini, and top with the shredded Gruyere cheese.

7. Sprinkle the crushed pork rinds over the top.

8. Bake for about 25 minutes, until the dish is bubbling and the top is nicely browned, and serve.

Nutrition: Calories: 324 Fat: 11.5g Fiber: 5.1g Carbohydrates: 2.2 g Protein: 5.1g

40. Olla Tapaha

Preparation time: 15 minutes

Cooking time: 25 minutes

Servings: 3

Ingredients:

- 2teaspoons canola oil
- 1red bell pepper, deveined and chopped
- 1shallot, chopped
- ½ cup celery rib, chopped
- ½ cup chayote, peeled and cubed
- 1pound (454 g) duck breasts, boneless, skinless, and chopped into small chunks
- 1½ cups vegetable broth
- ½ stick Mexican cinnamon
- 1thyme sprig
- 1rosemary sprig
- Sea salt and freshly ground black pepper, to taste

Directions:

1. Heat the canola oil in a soup pot (or clay pot) over a medium-high flame. Now, sauté the bell pepper,

shallot and celery until they have softened about 5 minutes.

2. Add the remaining ingredients and stir to combine. Once it starts boiling, turn the heat to simmer and partially cover the pot.

3. Let it simmer for 17 to 20 minutes or until thoroughly cooked. Enjoy!

Nutrition: calories: 230 fats: 9.6g protein: 30.5g carbs: 3.3g net carbs: 2.3g fiber: 1.0g

41. Leek and Pumpkin Turkey Stew

Preparation time: 20 minutes

Cooking time: 7 to 8 hours

Servings: 6

Ingredients:

- 3 tablespoons extra-virgin olive oil, divided
- 1pound (454 g) boneless turkey breast, cut into 1-inch pieces
- 1leek, thoroughly cleaned and sliced
- 2teaspoons minced garlic
- 2cups chicken broth
- 1cup coconut milk
- 2celery stalks, chopped
- 2cups diced pumpkin
- 1carrot, diced
- 2teaspoons chopped thyme
- Salt, for seasoning
- Freshly ground black pepper, for seasoning
- 1scallion, white and green parts, chopped, for garnish

Directions:

1. Lightly grease the insert of the slow cooker with 1tablespoon of the olive oil.

2. In a large skillet over medium-high heat, heat the remaining 2tablespoons of the olive oil. Add the turkey and sauté until browned, about 5 minutes.

3. Add the leek and garlic and sauté for an additional 3 minutes.

4. Transfer the turkey mixture to the insert and stir in the broth, coconut milk, celery, pumpkin, carrot, and thyme.

5. Cover and cook on low for 7 to 8 hours.

6. Season with salt and pepper.

7. Serve topped with the scallion.

Nutrition: calories: 357 fats: 27.0g protein: 21.0g carbs: 11.0g net carbs: 7.0g fiber: 4.0g

42. Indian Buttered Chicken

Preparation Time: 15 minutes

Cooking Time: 30 minutes

Servings: 4

Ingredients:

- 3 tablespoons unsalted butter
- 1medium yellow onion, chopped
- 2garlic cloves, minced
- 1teaspoon fresh ginger, minced
- 11/2pounds grass-fed chicken breasts, cut into 3/4-inch chunks
- 2tomatoes, chopped finely
- 1tablespoon garam masala
- 1teaspoon red chili powder
- 1teaspoon ground cumin
- Salt and ground black pepper, as required
- 1cup heavy cream
- 2tablespoons fresh cilantro, chopped

Directions:

1. In a wok, melt butter and sauté the onions for about 5–6 minutes.

2. Now, add in ginger and garlic and sauté for about 1minute.

3. Add the tomatoes and cook for about 2–3 minutes, crushing with the back of the spoon.

4. Stir in the chicken spices, salt, and black pepper, and cook for about 6–8 minutes or until the desired doneness of the chicken.

5. Put in the cream and cook for about 8–10 more minutes, stirring occasionally.

6. Garnish with fresh cilantro and serve hot.

Nutrition: Calories: 456 Fat: 14.1g Fiber: 10.5g Carbohydrates: 6.8 g Protein: 12.8 g

43. Chicken Parmigiana

Preparation Time: 15 minutes

Cooking Time: 25 minutes

Servings: 5

Ingredients:

- (6-ounce) grass-fed skinless, boneless chicken breasts
- 1large organic egg, beaten
- 1/2cup superfine blanched almond flour
- 1/4 cup Parmesan cheese, grated
- 1/2teaspoon dried parsley
- 1/2teaspoon paprika
- 1/2teaspoon garlic powder
- Salt and ground black pepper, as required
- 1/4 cup olive oil
- 1cup sugar-free tomato sauce
- 5 ounces' mozzarella cheese, thinly sliced
- 2tablespoons fresh parsley, chopped

Directions:

1. Preheat your oven to 375ºF.
2. Arrange one chicken breast between 2pieces of parchment paper.
3. With a meat mallet, pound the chicken breast into a 1/2-inch thickness

4. Repeat with the remaining chicken breasts.

5. Add the beaten egg into a shallow dish.

6. Place the almond flour, Parmesan, parsley, spices, salt, and black pepper in another shallow dish, and mix well.

7. Dip chicken breasts into the whipped egg and then coat with the flour mixture.

8. Heat the oil in a deep wok over medium-high heat and fry the chicken breasts for about 3 minutes per side.

9. The chicken breasts must be transferred onto a paper towel-lined plate to drain.

10. At the bottom of a casserole, place about 1/2cup of tomato sauce and spread evenly.

11. Arrange the chicken breasts over marinara sauce in a single layer.

12. Put sauce on top plus the mozzarella cheese slices.

13. Bake for about 20 minutes or until done completely.

14. Remove from the oven and serve hot with the garnishing of parsley.

Nutrition: Calories: 398 Fat: 15.1g Fiber: 9.4g Carbohydrates: 4.1g Protein: 15.1g

FISH AND SEAFOOD RECIPES

44. Pistachio Nut Salmon with Shallot Sauce

Preparation time:15 minutes

Cooking time: 30 minutes

Servings: 4

Ingredients:

- 4 salmon fillets
- ½ teaspoon pepper
- 1teaspoon salt
- ¼ cup mayonnaise
- ½ cup pistachios, chopped
- Sauce:
- 1shallot, chopped
- 2teaspoons lemon zest
- 1tablespoon olive oil
- A pinch of pepper
- 1cup heavy cream

Directions:

1. Preheat the oven to 375ºF (190ºC). Brush the salmon with mayonnaise and season with salt and pepper.

Coat with pistachios. Place in a lined baking dish, and bake, for 15 minutes.

2. Heat the olive oil in a saucepan, and sauté the shallots, for a few minutes. Stir in the rest of the sauce ingredients. Bring to a boil, and cook until thickened. Serve the salmon topped with the sauce.

Nutrition: calories: 564 fats: 47.0g protein: 34.0g carbs: 8.1g net carbs: 6.0g fiber: 2.1g

45. Spiced Jalapeno Bites with Tomato

Preparation Time: 10 minutes

Cooking Time: 0 minutes

Servings: 4

Ingredients:

- 1cup turkey ham, chopped
- 1/4 jalapeño pepper, minced
- 1/4 cup mayonnaise
- 1/3 tablespoon Dijon mustard
- 4 tomatoes, sliced
- Salt and black pepper, to taste
- 1tablespoon parsley, chopped

Directions:

1. In a bowl, mix the turkey ham, jalapeño pepper, mayo, mustard, salt, and pepper.

2. Spread out the tomato slices on four serving plates, then top each plate with a spoonful turkey ham mixture.

3. Serve garnished with chopped parsley.

Nutrition: Calories: 250 Fat: 14.1g Fiber: 3.7g Carbohydrates: 4.1g Protein: 18.9 g

46. Coconut Crab Cakes

Preparation Time: 20 minutes

Cooking Time: 25 minutes

Servings: 4

Ingredients:

- 1tablespoon of minced garlic
- 2pasteurized eggs
- 2teaspoons of coconut oil
- 3/4 cup of coconut flakes
- 3/4 cup chopped of spinach
- 1/4-pound crabmeat
- 1/4 cup of chopped leek
- 1/2cup extra virgin olive oil
- 1/2teaspoon of pepper
- 1/4 onion diced
- Salt

Directions:

1. Pour the crabmeat in a bowl, then add in the coconut flakes and mix well.
2. Whisk eggs in a bowl, then mix in leek and spinach.
3. Season the egg mixture with pepper, two pinches of salt, and garlic.
4. Then, pour the eggs into the crab and stir well.

5. Preheat a pan, heat extra virgin olive, and fry the crab evenly from each side until golden brown. Remove from pan and serve hot.

Nutrition: Calories: 254 Fat: 9.5g Fiber: 5.4g Carbohydrates: 4.1g Protein: 8.9g

SALADS RECIPES

47. Roasted Asparagus Salad

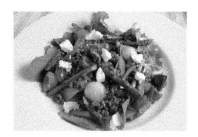

Preparation time: 15 minutes

Cooking time: 15 minutes

Servings: 5

Ingredients:

- 14 ounces (397 g) asparagus spears, trimmed
- 2tablespoons olive oil
- ½ teaspoon oregano
- ½ teaspoon rosemary
- Sea salt and freshly ground black pepper, to taste
- tablespoons mayonnaise
- 3 tablespoons sour cream
- 1tablespoon wine vinegar
- 1teaspoon fresh garlic, minced
- 1cup cherry tomatoes, halved

Directions:

1. In a lightly greased roasting pan, toss the asparagus with the olive oil, oregano, rosemary, salt, and black pepper.

2. Roast in the preheated oven at 425ºF (220ºC) for 13 to 15 minutes until just tender.

3. Meanwhile, in a mixing bowl, thoroughly combine the mayonnaise, sour cream, vinegar, and garlic; dress the salad and top with the cherry tomato halves.

4. Serve at room temperature. Bon appétit!

Nutrition: calories: 180 fat: 17.6g protein: 2.6g carbs: 4.5g net carbs: 2.5g fiber: 2.0g

48. Roasted Asparagus and Cherry Tomato Salad

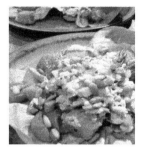

Preparation time: 15 minutes

Cooking time: 20 minutes

Servings: 3

Ingredients:

- 1pound (454 g) asparagus, trimmed
- ¼ teaspoon ground black pepper
- Flaky salt, to season
- 3 tablespoons sesame seeds
- 1tablespoon Dijon mustard
- ½ lime, freshly squeezed
- 3 tablespoons extra-virgin olive oil
- 2garlic cloves, minced
- 1tablespoon fresh tarragon, snipped
- 1cup cherry tomatoes, sliced

Directions:

1. Start by preheating your oven to 400ºF (205ºC). Spritz a roasting pan with nonstick cooking spray.

2. Roast the asparagus for about 13 minutes, turning the spears over once or twice. Sprinkle with salt, pepper, and sesame seeds; roast an additional 3 to 4 minutes.

3. To make the dressing, whisk the Dijon mustard, lime juice, olive oil, and minced garlic.

4. Chop the asparagus spears into bite-sized pieces and place them in a nice salad bowl. Add the tarragon and tomatoes to the bowl; gently toss to combine.

5. Dress your salad and serve at room temperature. Enjoy!

Nutrition: calories: 160 fat: 12.4g protein: 5.7g carbs: 6.2g net carbs: 2.2g fiber: 4.0g

DESSERT

49. Keto Blueberry Muffins

Preparation Time: 15 Minutes

Cooking Time: 1hour

Servings: 6

Ingredients:

- 1Stick/ 1/2cup/113 grams' butter
- 1teaspoon vanilla
- 8 tablespoons of fresh cheese
- 1cup coconut fibers
- 1/4 teaspoon Xanthan chewing gum
- 2teaspoons of baking soda
- 1/8 teaspoon cinnamon
- 1/2teaspoon salt
- Wet Ingredients
- 6 medium eggs
- 1/2Cup heavy cream
- 3/4 cup blueberries
- 4 teaspoons of coffee

Directions:

1. Mix butter, vanilla, and cream cheese in a bowl, add 2eggs, and beat the mixture again. Now add 1/3rd of

the dry ingredients and mix properly. Add 2more eggs and half of the dry ingredients and beat the mixture again.

2. Now add the last 2eggs and remaining of the dry ingredients and mix them properly. Finish the mixture by adding heavy cream and mix it properly until fully incorporated.

3. Add the berries and mix again. Now fill them in muffin containers and bake them for 30 minutes at 200 degrees C. Your muffins are ready.

Nutrition: Calories 234 Fat 12 Fiber 3 Carbs 2.3 Protein 19

50. Keto Oven-Baked Brie Cheese

Preparation Time: 15 Minutes

Cooking Time: 1hour

Servings: 8

Ingredients:

- 2cups brie or Camembert cheese
- 1tablespoon
- on olive oil
- 15 pecans or walnuts
- salt and pepper
- 1garlic clove
- 1tablespoon fresh rosemary

Directions:

1. Preheat the oven to 200C. Place the cheese on a baking tray lined with baking paper or in a small non-stick pan. Chop the garlic and roughly chop the nuts and herbs. Mix the three with olive oil. Add salt and pepper.

2. Put the walnut mixture over the cheese and bake for 10 minutes or until the cheese is lukewarm and soft and the nuts are toasted. Serve warm or tepid.

Nutrition: Calories 127 Fat 13 Fiber 3.8 Carbs 4 Protein 12

CONCLUSION

The keto diet is a low-carb, high-fat eating plan that changes the way your body uses energy. Normally, your body turns carbohydrates into glucose (a type of sugar and the main source of energy for your cells). But if you want to lose weight or improve certain medical conditions like diabetes, this diet might be for you. Some people think keto might even be beneficial for weight loss or specifically managing type 2 diabetes; researchers are studying these possibilities.

It's normal to feel hungry when you first start a low carbohydrate or "keto" diet because it takes time for your body to change and adjust. Your entire system begins to rely more and more on fat. There are two types of fat in your body: saturated and unsaturated. Saturated, or animal-based fats, increase LDL cholesterol (the bad kind) while unsaturated, or plant-based fats, do not. This is why consuming a diet high in animal based foods like red meat, butter and cheese increase your risk for heart disease.

What can you eat on the keto diet?

The keto diet also allows you to eat certain high-carb foods like fruit, vegetables, some grains (quinoa, amaranth and buckwheat) and dairy products like milk, yogurt and cheese (if you don't have an allergy). It's also a good idea to eat high-fiber foods, like spinach and avocado, since you'll need more fiber to keep your digestive tract running and absorb nutrients.

Is the ketogenic diet for everyone?

No. The keto diet is a very restrictive meal plan that requires careful monitoring. It can help control diabetes in some people, but it might not help in others. If you're considering trying this eating plan because of a specific medical condition, talk to your doctor first about whether it's safe for you and what type of monitoring you'll need. For people considering the keto diet, it's important to determine whether your goal is to treat a specific health condition or lose weight, and how serious you are about this goal.

As in any other diet, if you take our word for it, make sure it is working for you before investing your time and money.

Lightning Source UK Ltd.
Milton Keynes UK
UKHW022016190421
382278UK00003B/614